COSTOCHONDRITIS

ALL QUESTIONS ON COSTOCHONDRITIS
ANSWERED

DR. J. SIMON

Contents

INTRODUCTION

The area of inflamed cartilage where the upper ribs join the sternum in cases of osteochondritis is referred to as the "costosternal junction". Inflammatory-related chest discomfort and soreness can occasionally mimic the signs of more serious illnesses, such as heart-related conditions. Costochondritis symptoms can be distressing, despite the fact that they are typically benign and moderate.

While the exact cause of costochondritis is frequently unknown, it is believed to be related to cartilage wear and tear, excessive physical activity, or viral infections. This is a condition that primarily affects women over the age of forty.

Costochondritis does not result in more severe health problems, although its symptoms might be uncomfortable and interfere with daily activities. It is essential to seek medical evaluation in order to rule out other potential causes of chest pain and to determine the best course of treatment. Treatment typically entails lifestyle changes and pain management strategies to alleviate discomfort.

CHAPTER ONE

The Meaning of Chondritis

Costochondritis is the name for a non-serious inflammation of the cartilage at the costosternal junction, which connects a rib to the sternum, the breastbone. The symptoms of this sickness include pain and discomfort in the chest, especially where the upper ribs join the sternum. Notwithstanding the occasionally concerning discomfort, osteochondritis is usually a benign and self-limiting condition.

Costosternal, costovertebral, or costosternal joint inflammation is thought to be the cause of costochondritis, while the exact cause is frequently unknown. It can affect people of all ages, though it is more commonly seen in adults, and often has no apparent reason.

As osteochondritis can resemble the symptoms of more serious conditions including heart difficulties or other types of chest pain, anybody experiencing discomfort in their chest should see a doctor. In order to rule out other potential causes of chest discomfort, a physical examination, a review of the patient's medical history, and occasionally imaging tests are utilized in the diagnosing process.

Despite the fact that costochondritis alone does not result in long-term issues or damage to the heart or other organs, it is imperative to manage symptoms and seek the assistance of a trained medical practitioner to reduce discomfort and offer relief. Common methods of treating discomfort include nonsteroidal anti-inflammatory drugs (NSAIDs) and lifestyle changes that lessen stress on the chest area.

Motives and Risk Factors

While the exact cause of costochondritis is often unknown, the condition is generally considered benign and self-limiting. On the other hand, costochondritis may develop as a result of several factors and potential triggers. Among the common causes and warning indicators are:

Trauma or Injury:

A blow to the chest or other trauma can increase costochondritis by causing inflammation in the costosternal, costovertebral, or costosternal joints.

Recurrent Stress:

Repetitive arm and upper body movements and activities may raise the risk of developing costochondritis, especially if they place strain or stress on the chest wall.

Physical strain:

Prolonged, strong upper body movements, hard lifting, and intense physical activity can all exacerbate the inflammation of the costosternal junction.

Viral infections:

Evidence exists that some viral infections, particularly those of the respiratory system, are linked to the development of costochondritis. It is thought that the viral infection may lead to cartilage inflammation, albeit the exact mechanism is yet unclear.

Jointessential infections:

Rarely, bacterial or fungal infections affecting the costovertebral, costosternal, or costosternal joints can cause inflammation and costochondritis.

Conditions Resulting from an Autoimmune Reaction:

Two autoimmune illnesses that may increase the risk of joint inflammation, including inflammation in the chest wall, are rheumatoid arthritis and ankylosing spondylitis.

Joint Stress Is Caused by Poor Posture:

Slouching or rounding the shoulders, especially when sitting or standing for extended periods of time, can put tension on the costosternal junction and could make inflammation worse.

The Costosternum Syndrome:

Those who have costosternal syndrome, a condition characterized by ongoing irritation of the costovertebral or costosternal joints, may be at an increased risk of developing costochondritis.

Gender and age are risk factors for costochondritis, with a higher incidence of the disease in women than in men. People over 40 are more likely to have the disorder. Individuals who have already sustained chest injuries, participate in repetitive activities, or have certain medical conditions may also be at a higher risk.

It's important to note that costochondritis is typically diagnosed as an exclusion diagnosis, requiring further testing to rule out other potential causes of chest pain, such as cardiac issues. Seeking medical help as soon as possible is essential for someone experiencing severe or persistent chest discomfort, as it allows for an accurate diagnosis and treatment plan.

The primary symptoms of costochondritis are chest discomfort and soreness, which can vary in intensity and duration. Symptoms of costochondritis typically include:

Chest pain:

Chest pain, often characterized as a severe or excruciating feeling, is the primary symptom. The pain is typically located in the costosternal or costovertebral joints, which attach the upper ribs to the sternum or spine.

Sensitivity

Tenderness is brought on by applying pressure to the costosternal, costovertebral, or costosternal joints. Placing pressure on the affected area may exacerbate or reproduce the pain.

Motion Makes Pain Worse:

The chest pain that is frequently associated with costochondritis can intensify with specific movements or activities. Sneezing, coughing, deep breathing, and exercises involving a lot of movement in the upper body are a few things that can make discomfort worse.

Pain Control during Sleep:

Resting or avoiding activities that exacerbate the discomfort can help relieve it. Unlike heart-related chest pain, costochondritis pain is usually not brought on by exercise.

Throat Pain that Shoots Up:

While chest pain is the primary symptom of costochondritis, arm discomfort is also a possible symptom for certain individuals. Sometimes, this could be confused with heart attack symptoms, such as chest pain.

Not Able to Breathe:

Sometimes, people with costochondritis feel as though their breathing is difficult or their chest is constricted. But this isn't caused by a heart or lung problem; rather, it's the associated chest ache.

It's important to keep in mind that while costochondritis can cause excruciating chest discomfort, the heart and other major organs are unaffected. Though the symptoms can be distressing, it's crucial to see a doctor to rule out more serious conditions including heart issues or other causes of chest pain.

It is imperative that someone experiencing severe or chronic chest discomfort receives quick medical attention, especially if there are accompanying symptoms such as nausea, shortness of breath, or pain moving down the arm, in order to rule out other possible causes and ensure effective care.

Recognition and Medical Evaluation

A thorough medical evaluation is typically necessary for the diagnosis of costochondritis in order to rule out other potential causes of chest discomfort and assess the condition's characteristic symptoms. The following are common steps and considerations for costochondritis diagnosis:

Background Information on Health:

The medical professional will take a complete medical history and ask about the kind, duration, and intensity of the chest pain. They could inquire about any recent trauma, repetitive motion injuries, or respiratory infections.

Physical Evaluation:

A physical examination looks for pain or edema in the chest, as well as any signs of inflammation around the costosternal, costovertebral, or costosternal joints. The medical expert may apply pressure to certain areas to mimic or exacerbate the discomfort.

Throw Away Heart-Related Causes:

Because chest pain can have a variety of causes, it is important to rule out cardiac issues. An electrocardiogram, or EKG, may be performed by the medical practitioner to assess heart function. If necessary, further cardiac testing may be requested.

Imaging Tests:

Chest X-rays and other imaging tests can occasionally be carried out to rule out further potential causes of chest pain, such as lung issues or fractures. X-rays help rule out other conditions but typically do not identify costochondritis.

Laboratory Tests:

Blood tests can be performed to search for signs of inflammation or illness. Elevated levels of inflammatory markers may lend credence to the costochondritis diagnosis.

Additional Diagnostic Methods:

In certain situations, additional diagnostic tests like computed tomography (CT) scans or magnetic resonance imaging (MRI) may be required to further evaluate the chest and rule out additional potential causes of pain.

Standards for Diagnosis:

To diagnose costochondritis, a combination of clinical features, physical examination findings, and ruling out other reasons are commonly employed. Since there are no specific clinical or laboratory signs for costochondritis, diagnosis might be challenging.

Individuals experiencing discomfort in the chest should see a doctor, particularly if the pain is severe, persistent, or accompanied by other concerning symptoms. Despite the fact that costochondritis is usually a benign and self-limiting condition, a correct diagnosis is necessary for the best course of treatment and to rule out more serious conditions that may require other therapies.

CHAPTER TWO

Techniques for Counseling

Symptom alleviation and discomfort management are the main objectives of treatment for costochondritis. Despite the fact that costochondritis normally goes away on its own, there are a number of ways to improve overall health and reduce pain in those who are experiencing chest pain. The typical approaches to treating costochondritis are as follows:

Drugs for the Relief of Pain:

Two advantages of utilizing nonsteroidal anti-inflammatory drugs (NSAIDs), such as ibuprofen or naproxen, are pain alleviation and reduced inflammation. These medications usually provide good symptom management for costochondritis.

Heat or Cold Therapy:

Applying heat or ice to the affected area might help reduce pain and inflammation. Use heat pads or compresses for comfort.

Take a break and avoid activities that set them off:

Resting and avoiding activities that irritate chest pain can help hasten the healing process. It is advised that people modify their daily routines in order to alleviate the strain on their chest.

Physical Therapy:

Physical therapy may be suggested in order to strengthen muscles, enhance flexibility, and correct posture. Certain exercises can help prevent recurrence and promote overall chest health.

Techniques for Reducing Pain:

By practicing deep breathing exercises, relaxation techniques, and other pain management strategies, people can manage their pain and lower their stress levels. This may help patients manage their discomfort and maybe reduce their symptoms.

Changing Position:

Especially whether sitting or standing, good posture can help prevent tension on the chest wall and reduce the likelihood of repeated pain.

Over-the-Counter Topical Painkillers:

Topical analgesic creams or patches containing ingredients like menthol or camphor can provide localized pain relief.

Prescription Medicines:

Sometimes a doctor will prescribe stronger painkillers or muscle relaxants if the patient has severe or persistent pain.

Counseling and stress reduction:

Counseling or stress management techniques could be beneficial, especially if stress aggravates symptoms.

Analyzing the Contributing Elements:

If costochondritis is associated with an underlying illness, such as rheumatoid arthritis or ankylosing spondylitis, treating that condition is necessary for long-term symptom relief.

For anyone experiencing chest pain, seeing a medical practitioner is essential to getting a proper diagnosis and course of treatment. Despite the fact that costochondritis is mostly benign, it's crucial to ensure that symptoms are properly controlled and rule out any other potential causes of chest pain. If conservative measures fail to relieve the discomfort or if it worsens, more evaluation might be necessary.

Factors Related to Lifestyle to Consider

Lifestyle decisions are crucial in managing and averting the recurrence of costochondritis. Modifying particular lifestyle choices and habits can enhance overall chest health and reduce the likelihood of worsening symptoms. The following aspects of lifestyle are crucial for those who have costochondritis:

Maintain Proper Posture:

Improving posture, especially when sitting or standing, can help lessen the tension on the chest area. Avoid slouching and maintain a neutral spine posture.

Cozy Workspace:

If you work a desk job, make sure the area where you work is ergonomic. Pick a chair with adequate lumbar support, position your computer at eye level, and take breaks to stretch and move about.

Gentle Exercise:

Engage in low-impact exercises that improve your overall health, flexibility, and strength. Gentle exercises such as yoga, swimming, or walking may be beneficial.

Avoid doing a lot of hard lifting:

Steer clear of activities that need a lot of upper body strength, such as heavy lifting. If lifting is necessary, do it cautiously so as not to put undue tension on your chest muscles.

Breathing Methods:

Practice deep breathing to expand lung capacity and reduce strain in the chest. Particularly useful for managing stress and anxiety are breathing exercises.

Managing Body Weight:

Maintaining a healthy weight helps alleviate pressure on the chest area and enhance overall musculoskeletal health.

Methods for Stress Reduction:

Incorporate stress-reduction tactics, such as mindfulness, meditation, or relaxation methods, into your regular routine. Excessive stress can exacerbate conditions and cause strained muscles.

The Appropriate Sleep Position

Make sure your chest is properly supported as you sleep. Using supportive pillows and mattresses can help you maintain optimal spine alignment.

Avoid wearing tight garments.

Wearing tight clothing, particularly around the chest, may exacerbate discomfort. Wear loose-fitting, comfortable clothing to lessen the tension on the costosternal joints.

Regular Extension:

Regularly incorporate stretches into your routine to maintain the flexibility of your upper body and chest. Stretching helps prevent tense muscles and reduce the risk of injury.

Optimal Nutrition:

Maintain a diet rich in the nutrients essential to the overall health of your musculoskeletal system, while also keeping it well-balanced. Adequate consumption of vitamins and minerals promotes the healing process.

Consuming lots of water

To keep your general health and your muscles and joints functioning at their peak, make sure you are getting enough water into your body.

It's important to customize these lifestyle issues based on one's preferences, activities, and health. Consultation with a physician or physical therapist may provide targeted guidance on lifestyle adjustments tailored to the unique needs of individuals with costochondritis.

When to Seek Medical Assistance

Despite the fact that costochondritis is mostly benign and self-limiting, there are situations in which patients should see a doctor straight immediately. If you experience severe symptoms or other warning signs in addition to unexplained chest pain or discomfort, you should definitely seek medical attention. You should consult a doctor if any of the following situations apply to your costochondritis:

Torrential Chest Pain:

If your acute or intense chest pain does not go away with rest or over-the-counter pain medication, get emergency medical attention.

Radiating pain to the arm or jaw:

If pain travels from the chest down the jaw, down the left arm, or into the back, it is imperative to seek emergency medical attention. These signs might point to a more severe cardiac issue.

Shortness of Breath:

Any dyspnea or breathing difficulties caused on by chest pain should be evaluated immediately. This may indicate a more serious issue with the heart or lungs.

CHAPTER THREE

Experiencing nausea or vomiting:

Chest pain that is accompanied by vomiting or nausea may be a sign of a cardiac event or another dangerous sickness that needs to be treated immediately.

Sweating or dizziness:

If you experience lightheadedness, fainting, or heavy perspiration in addition to chest pain, you should call emergency services as these symptoms may point to a medical emergency.

New or Increased Symptoms:

In the event that you have been diagnosed with costochondritis and your symptoms are either new or worsening, or if your symptoms have changed, it is recommended that you consult a healthcare provider for a reevaluation.

Prolonged Symptoms:

If your chest discomfort does not improve with rest, medication, and lifestyle modifications, consult a healthcare provider to see if imaging tests or additional evaluation are necessary.

History of Heart Disease:

When seeking treatment for chest discomfort, people with a history of heart disease or other cardiovascular risk factors should exercise extra caution.

Even though chest pain is often related to costochondritis, doctors perform a comprehensive procedure to rule out other potential causes, such as heart conditions, respiratory issues, or gastrointestinal diseases. If you are unclear or if your symptoms are severe, do not hesitate to call for emergency medical assistance or visit the nearest emergency room for an assessment. Chest pain should always be carefully treated. A prompt medical evaluation ensures the appropriate diagnosis and treatment plan.

Long-Term Prospects and Coping Strategies

The prognosis is generally positive because costochondritis is a self-limiting condition that frequently improves with time and appropriate care. The majority of people experience symptom relief with conservative treatments. Nonetheless, coping strategies can further enhance a person with costochondritis's general quality of life:

Frequent Monitoring

Continue seeing your doctor for routine check-ups to discuss any changes in your symptoms and to monitor your recovery. The course of treatment may need to be adjusted.

Modifications to Lifestyle:

You should regularly practice stress management techniques, limit activities that exacerbate symptoms, and maintain appropriate posture, to name a few lifestyle improvements.

Exercise and physical therapy:

The muscles that surround the chest can be strengthened and made more flexible by regular low-impact exercise and physical therapy. This could reduce the chance of developing costochondritis in the future.

Techniques for Reducing Pain:

Learn and use pain management practices, such as mindfulness, deep breathing exercises, and relaxation techniques, to control pain and reduce stress.

Understanding and Awareness:

Find out everything you can about the causes and treatments of costochondritis. Making informed decisions about your health may be made easier if you are aware of the ailment.

Flexible Work Environment:

Consider modifying your workstation or implementing ergonomic practices if you do tasks at work that increase your chance of experiencing chest pain.

Helping Mechanism:

Create a support system by reaching out to others who have experienced similar difficulties. Support groups and internet forums provide a space for people to share their experiences and coping strategies.

Selecting a Healthier Way of Living:

Maintain your health by prioritizing a balanced diet, regular exercise, and adequate sleep. These components promote overall wellness and might help with symptom management.

Exercises for Pacing:

Take it slow and pay attention to your physical activity. Pay attention to your body's signals and don't overdo it to prevent hurting the chest area.

Engaging with the Healthcare Professional:

Keep in touch with your healthcare provider on a frequent basis. If your symptoms change, or if you have any concerns, get in touch with someone straight immediately so that your condition can be properly addressed.

It's important to keep in mind that while costochondritis normally improves over time, flare-ups may still occur on occasion. People can effectively manage their symptoms and lead fulfilling lives by adopting and understanding coping methods. If after using these strategies your symptoms worsen or persist, consult your physician for further evaluation and guidance.

CONCLUSION

In summary, costochondritis is an inflammatory disease that affects the cartilage in the chest, causing pain and tightness in the area. Although the exact cause is often unknown, the condition is usually considered benign and self-limiting.

Long-term prognosis for those with costochondritis is favorable since most patients discover that conservative measures including rest, medication, and lifestyle changes can reduce symptoms. Knowing your triggers, maintaining regular check-ins with medical providers, and continuing self-care practices all contribute to effective therapy.

To treat costochondritis, a multimodal approach that incorporates physical therapy, stress management, and maintaining a healthy lifestyle is required. Building a support system, communicating openly with medical professionals, and learning about the condition are all necessary for improving overall well-being.

Chest discomfort sufferers should seek medical attention as soon as possible, particularly if their symptoms are severe, persistent, or accompanied by other concerning symptoms. Even though costochondritis alone is typically not associated with potentially fatal consequences, a clear diagnosis ensures appropriate care and rules out other potential causes of chest pain.

Costochondritis can be managed and a high quality of life preserved by individuals who adopt a proactive, comprehensive approach to health and consistently practice self-care. Remember that each person's experience is different, and consulting with medical professionals is necessary for individualized and effective treatment.

THE END